Meal Prep

65+ Meal Prep Recipes Cookbook – Step By Step Meal Prepping Guide For Rapid Weight Loss

John Carter

Introduction

I want to thank you and congratulate you for downloading the book, *"Meal Prep."*

Obesity remains one of the biggest health problems in the world. Obesity is a result of wrong food choices coupled with a sedentary lifestyle. The food that people eat these days is filled with sugars, fats and chemicals. Right through from junk to processed foods, people end up consuming elements that their bodies are incapable of digesting thereby leading to health complications.

Add to it the stress of everyday life, and a lack of motivation to take up physical activities, it's not surprising that people pile on pounds. The need of the hour therefore is to remedy the situation through the application of a simple diet and meal prepping routine that can offset weight gain.

Meal prepping refers to preparing a meal in advance. As you know, most people are pressed for time and end up ordering food from restaurants. This directly contributes towards weight gain and can lead to obesity. But just with a little pre-planning and prepping, people will be able to tackle this issue.

In this book, we look at the simple things you can do to prep for meals in advance and get you started on a few simple recipes that can be prepped in advance.

Thanks again for downloading this book, I hope you enjoy it!

TABLE OF CONTENTS

Bonus: FREE Report Reveals The Secrets To Lose Weight

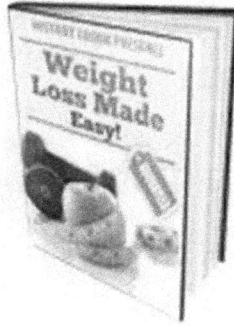

Weight loss doesn't happen from dieting only. Diets are short term solutions to shed extra weight. Diets do not work in the long term because people hate being on a diet (it's ok, you can admit that here). The only long term solution for permanent weight loss is to create new eating habits. This doesn't mean that chocolate will never pass your lips again, but it does mean looking after yourself and watching what you eat...

You can lose weight when you have the right reasons and motivation, and a part of this guide is to help you to find the motivation you need to change your weight...

Click Here to Get This Guid For FREE

Chapter 1: What Is Meal Prep? Why Is It Important?

In this first chapter, we will look at the meaning of prepping meals, why it is important to do so and how you can prep meals in advance.

What is meal prepping?

Preparation takes center stage when it comes to enhancing good health through the application of a healthy diet. Preparing in advance helps you remain ready to cook the meals for the day. Meal prepping is a simple concept that can provide you with multiple benefits. It refers to preparing for your meals in advance so that you can save time, effort and energy.

Meal prepping is a practice where you prepare simple meals in advance. These can pertain to your breakfasts, lunches and dinners. It is a theory that can be a big help, especially if you are trying to lose weight or improve your health. This, in fact, is especially important in this day and age where every other person is trying to lose weight and develop a lean body. It is now seen as a great way to achieve good health. You do not have to worry about a time crunch or ordering takeaways every other day. Just by preparing in advance, you can take steps towards enhancing good health.

Meal prepping can mean different things to different people, as there are many different ways to do it. Some prefer to prepare the ingredients alone while others prepare entire meals. What you choose to do is entirely up to you and you can pick whatever suits your needs.

Why is meal prep important?

It is extremely important to prep for a meal in advance, as you will be able to cut down on cooking time. More importantly, you will be in a position to prepare a great tasting meal. Here are some of the advantages of prepping for a meal in advance:

Health

One of the main advantages of prepping for a meal in advance is that you will be able to achieve good health. Take away foods are one of health's biggest enemies. Even if you end up eating at a "healthy joint" you will still be subjecting yourself to chemicals and toxins that are bad for your body. It would, therefore, be a good idea to prep for a meal in advance. You will also be determined to prepare healthier meals for yourself. You will make it a point to prep for salads, soups, stews etc. in a bid to improve your health.

Metabolism

Prepping foods in advance can help you enhance your metabolism. When you marinate foods, you end up encouraging them to tenderize and release their goodness. Consuming the same will help you enhance your bodily functions. Your body will not have to put in as much effort to digest the food and can break down the complex food molecules much easily.

Save time

The next important advantage is that you will be able to save time. As we know, most of us lead busy lives and end up sacrificing our health in a bid to meet deadlines and commitments. But through prepping, you will be able to save time and effort. You can still enjoy elaborate meals that are rich in flavor and nutrition. You can stave off the need to order food from outside and prepare your own delicious and nutritious meals at home. Just through prepping, you can cut down on as much as 70% of your cooking time. The same time can be directed towards fulfilling more enjoyable activities.

Cost effective

Prepping for meals can be quite cost effective. You will not have to spend as much on takeaways and eating at restaurants. By prepping, you will also not end up wasting food and, in turn, can use this extra money to buy healthy ingredients. You will also find it convenient to prepare your own condiments such as sauces and dips and save money on these items.

These form some of the advantages of prepping your meals in advance but the benefits are not limited to these. You will come face to face with the rest, as and when you start prepping your meals.

How to prep meals?

Imagine returning home after a tiring day's work and hunching over the table to cut vegetables or meats. You will not feel like doing it and end up ordering a take away. But just by prepping for a meal, you will be able to avoid this situation and prepare a healthy meal.

Prepping meals helps in many different ways. You don't have to worry about doing everything at the last minute, as everything will be in place, requiring only a little assembly. Meal prepping is fairly simple and does not require you to put in too much effort. Just with a little planning, you will be able to prep meals that can last for a week or as much as up to 6 months. But you will have to adopt a few simple steps towards the same in order to prep the ingredients in the correct manner.

Planning

The very first step is to plan for the prep. This might sound strange since prepping itself stands for planning. However, in order to prep for an entire week, month or even 6 months, you will have to first plan everything out.

If you are new to food preparation, then you might have to take it a little slowly. Trying to do too much at once can intimidate you. Start by making a list of the foods and other items required to prep for a meal. This includes groceries, condiments, meal boxes, cling film, aluminum foil etc. The list has to be as comprehensive as possible so that it becomes easy for you to buy all of it at the supermarket.

Next up, write down a meal plan for a week or two. If you are just starting out then you can write it down for just 3 or 4 days. Prepare a menu for breakfast, lunch and dinner. Write down exactly what you will be making including the recipes for each of the meals. If you have a few standard recipes that you are good at preparing, then stick with these. But remember; pick those recipes that are not easily going to spoil. You might have to preserve them for a long time and must, therefore, pick whatever lasts at least a month or that can be frozen.

Prepping

The next step is to prep for the meals. Prepping refers to keeping everything ready for the meal or preparing the meal and storing it.

Try to pick different recipes so that you don't get bored with it or find it monotonous. A good idea is for you to stick to known recipes for the first couple of months before experimenting with different tastes.

Timing

Timing is crucial for your prepping. When you time the prepping, you know exactly how much needs to be prepared and set aside. You will also know exactly how long the prepared meals will last. There are no set rules for when you can and cannot prep for a meal. You can prepare for a meal the previous night or 10 nights in advance. You will have to judge as to how long it will last and how much time it will cut down on your cooking time.

As a rule, it will be important to prep for a big meal well in advance. That way, you will have time to prep properly and not leave out any crucial ingredient of the meal. With time, you will know exactly when to prep a meal and how in advance you will need to do so.

Cooking

It is important to note that prepping does not mean you can avoid cooking. You will still have to cook a meal in order to consume it. Say, for example, you plan to make roast ribs. You can prep this by adding it to a Ziploc bag along with seasoning and place it in the fridge. When you are ready to cook, you simply remove it from the bag and add to the oven or grill.

The basic idea of prepping is to reduce the time taken during cooking and this is especially important if you have an elaborate meal to cook. You might have to cut vegetables, grind pastes, extract juices etc. all of which can take up time. You will find it much easier to cook up the meal if all of these are prepared in advance.

You will also be in a position to prepare a lovely meal that tastes great with minimal effort.

Chapter 2: Meal Prepping Essentials

In the previous chapter, we looked at the meaning and importance of meal prepping. In this chapter, we will look at the essentials of meal prepping. When it comes to prepping for a meal, you will need a few basic items that are as follows:

Containers

First, you will require containers in which to place the prepped ingredients. Containers can be of any shape and size depending on your needs. If you are prepping for a big family then choose large containers that can hold a lot more of the ingredients. It would be ideal to buy containers that are microwave safe. Ensure that all the containers are BPA free. Try to have separate containers for vegetables and meats as mixing them can cause the flavors to mingle and interfere with the taste of the meal. If you are keen on prepping several meals at a time, then consider buying the containers at wholesale stores that provide you with discounts. But try not to compromise on quality and go for unbreakable, airtight containers that are easy to wash up.

Bottles

Next, you will need bottles to store broths, stocks, juices etc. Try to buy bottles that are hardy and long lasting. You can buy whatever quantity you need depending on how much you think will be prepare in advance. The bottles should fit in the fridge or freezer. They should be BPA free and also free from odor.

Cling film

You will require cling film to cover some of the bowls or boxes containing the prepped ingredients. Buy good quality cling film that can serve multiple purposes. Have 2 or 3 spare rolls that are easily available whenever you need them.

Aluminum foil

You will need aluminum foil to cover or wrap the prepped ingredients. This is especially important if you want something to remain warm. Using foil can also ensure tenderizing of meats and vegetables. Buy good quality foil and have 2 or 3 spare rolls in stock.

Ziploc bags

Ziploc bags are a must when you wish to prep for a meal. Ziploc bags not only seal in moisture and flavor but also prevent the foods from going bad. They are also easy to store in the fridge or freezer and take up far less space when compared to containers.

Now that you know what you need to buy in order to store the prepped ingredients, we will look at how you can prep some of the different elements of a meal.

Vegetables and fruits

It is extremely important for you to prep your vegetables and fruits well in advance. Vegetables are extremely important for your body. You have to consume at least 5 different types of vegetables on a daily basis. The best way to prep is by washing them thoroughly before peeling and chopping. Once done, transfer them to containers that are clean and dry. The same extends to fruits. You must wash and chop them before adding to containers. If you do not wish to chop the vegetables or fruits just before cooking, then you can wash, peel and add them to Ziploc bags. Store the bags in the freezer if you wish to use them much later or in the fridge, if you plan on using them very soon.

Meats

Meats are one of the most important parts of a meal. They are rich in protein and can help build leaner muscles. There are many types of meats to choose from and you can pick whatever you are comfortable with. The best way to prep meats is by first cleaning them thoroughly by rinsing them. You must try to get rid of as many germs from the meat as possible. Once done, chop it to the desired size and add to the containers. If you wish to marinate the meats, then first prepare the marinade and add to the container before adding in the meat. It will be best to pick containers for wet marinades and Ziploc bags for dry rubs.

Carbohydrates

Carbohydrates are generally regarded as villains considering the effect they can have on the body. However, not all carbs are bad carbs and it is essential for your body to eat a minimum amount in order to carry out basic activities. There are many sources of carbohydrates but is best to choose whole grains such as quinoa, wheat, barley etc. Switching up white rice with brown rice can also help you tackle some of the issues associated with carbohydrate intake. To prep carbs, you have to ensure that everything is dry as even a little moisture can end up spoiling your ingredients. If you are mixing them with vegetables then try to dry the vegetables before adding in the carbs.

Liquids

When it comes to storing liquids, you have to choose airtight bottles that are sturdy and spill proof. You can store many types of liquids including stocks, sauces, broths, soups, stews etc. Bone broth is a great liquid to have in your pantry, as it is full of healthy nutrients. It is also quite versatile and can be added to prepare a variety of meals. You can easily prepare the broth at home by adding bones and water to a cooker and setting it on manual for 40 minutes. Wait for it to cool down before discarding the bones and straining the liquid into bottles.

Sides

No meal is complete without sides and so you must prep for them in order to have a complete meal. Right from pickles to relishes, you can prepare sides in advance and store them in airtight containers. Place them in the fridge if you use them on a daily basis. If you wish to store a large batch then add it to the freezer.

Snacks

You can prep and store snacks the same way as you would regular meals. You can store chopped vegetables such as carrots, beetroots, celery sticks etc. and add them to airtight containers. You can also pack dips to go along with them.

Meals

If you wish to store entire meals in containers then it will take a lot more effort from your end, but is well worth it considering you won't have to cook after a busy day. Here are some pointers to help you out

If you plan on storing food for a week then ensure that it contains ingredients that can last that long. You can refer to a chart that tells you what foods can be stored for a week without spoiling.

If you wish to store cooked meals in the fridge then ensure you consume them within 3 days. You have to add them to the freezer if you plan on consuming them after 3 days.

Always check the food by first smelling it. If it does not smell good, then discard it. Some foods can smell good but taste bad so eat a small quantity first to determine whether the meal is good enough to be consumed.

Try to label your foods with dates so that you know when the food was prepared.

Do not put a used spoon or fork into the food and then store it. This will spoil the food. The same extends to using your fingers.

Chapter 3: Simple Meal Prep Ideas to Save Time and Effort

Eating the same foods over and over again can get extremely monotonous. In order to fix this issue, you can adopt a few simple ideas that can help you prep simple yet delicious meals.

3 in 1

If you want to have a different type of meat every night then you can marinate them in 3 different ways. All you need is a large glass tray (or any tray) and some aluminum foil. Line the tray with the aluminum foil. Make two partitions by flattening out the foil. Add the meat to the tray so that you have three equal parts. Add three different sauces or marinades to the sections and toss in your chopped meat. Cover with cling film or aluminum foil and place in the fridge. You can use them as and when you like without getting bored.

Smoothie muffins

A great hack to store your smoothies for a longer time is to freeze them in muffin molds. All you have to do is prepare the smoothies and add them to the molds and place in the freezer. All you need to do is allow them to thaw naturally or add to the Instant Pot for 5 minutes.

Timing

A good way to cook many different vegetables at once is by mixing 3 or 4 that have the same cooking time. For example, beans and cauliflower take about the same time to cook and so can be added together to the same container. Similarly, add 3 or

4 vegetables with similar cooking times so that you can cook them with ease.

Portions

One good way of staving off overeating is by packing the right portions. This means that you pack the exact amount of food that you will be consuming per meal. Buy smaller boxes and pack in the measured meal. For example, buy a box that can contain just 4 pretzels or 3 cookies. That way, you will know how many to eat and stop when the quota has been reached.

Breakfast

Breakfast is the most important meal of the day. You have to consume a healthy breakfast in order to remain fit and active throughout the day. A good idea is to prepare oatmeal jars by adding in different fruits and nuts to each jar. That way, you will not get bored and have easy access to a healthy breakfast. The correct method to prep it would be to add the cereal at the bottom, about a quarter of the way up, followed by the chopped fruits. You can also sprinkle some nuts and seeds on top.

Prep for juices

Many times, we end up adding in too many ingredients to the blender or juicer and are left with extra-large helpings of juices and smoothies. In order to avoid this, it will be a good idea to prep the exact number of fruits that will be used per smoothie or juice. Cut it up and add it to containers so that you can easily add it to the blender or juicer.

Salads

It is advisable for you to consume as many salads as possible in order to enhance good health. You do not have to always assemble a salad from scratch and can prepare them well in advance. A salad jar will make for a great idea and can be carried anywhere. A typical jar can contain as many different vegetables as you would like to consume. Start by adding the dressing at the bottom followed by beans followed by vegetables and topped off with the leaves. You can empty the jar into a bowl just before consuming the salad and find the dressing on top.

Spiralizer

The spiralizer is a great gadget to have in your kitchen. You can use it to spiralize vegetables and add to containers. The spiralizer can be used to spiralize different types of vegetables regardless of their rigidity. In fact, it will be best to use it to spiralize hard vegetables such as beetroots and carrots, which are otherwise tough to chop. Stacking the vegetables on top of each other will make for a colorful sight and encourage you to cook more.

Chapter 4: Mistakes to Avoid While Prepping Meals

It is obvious that you will end up making a few mistakes when you start out with prepping meals. In order to help you with this, here are some common mistakes that people make and how you can avoid them.

Overdoing it

Many people make the mistake of preparing too much in advance. You will only end up wasting food if you do so and must, therefore, plan it out correctly. If you follow a few basic rules you will be able to cook the right amount without worrying about wasting food. Here is a step-by-step guide to follow.

- Plan everything out in advance. Right from the amount of food to be prepped to the type of meals to be prepped and the number of ingredients to prep etc.

- You have to calculate the calorie intake of every member of your family so that you can prep the meals accordingly. Ask them to give you a number so that you know how much to prep

- You will have to indulge in a certain degree of trial and error to know exactly how much needs to be prepped for your family. Observe for a week, or even a month, to know the exact figure

- Think of all the money and ingredients you will be wasting by cooking too much food. You can save on it just by prepping for the meals in advance

- If in case you end up with too much food then check to see if it can be kept in the freezer for the next day. That way, you will at least be able to put some of it to good use

- Always account for any increase in the quantity of the ingredients through swelling or absorption of water. This mostly happens with beans, chickpeas etc. You have to prep these bearing in mind the final quantity they will produce

Under doing it

Another mistake to avoid is cooking too little. Remember that prepping not only helps you save money and time but also gives you an opportunity to achieve good health. You have to, therefore, plan the meals in such a way that you are able to satisfy your hunger at every meal. If you fail to do so then chances are high you will end up consuming unhealthy snacks to make up for the deficit. Remember that everybody goes through this at the very beginning and must take away lessons from the same. Observe yourself through the course of a week and write down how much food you prepped, how much was consumed and how much was wasted. That will give you a good idea of how much needs to be prepared for the next week.

Monotony

You must make food as interesting as possible and avoid monotony at all costs. Eating the same type of foods can make it extremely boring for you. You have to, therefore, plan your meals in such a way that you have the chance to eat something different every single day. You do not have to change up the entire meal and only modify the seasoning. Try switching up your barbecue sauce for some Sriracha or your Italian seasoning for some Indian curry powder. Avoid over seasoning the ingredients as that can make the meal taste bad.

Relying on ready-made condiments

Some people resort to shortcuts and end up using store bought sauces and condiments. This is not the right way of going about it as you will end up adding unwanted sugars to your body. You must aim at making your own condiments using fresh ingredients. Once you have the recipe you will find it easy to prepare them and not rely on store bought stuff.

Foods you dislike

Some people end up prepping for meals they dislike. Although it might sound strange, people end up prepping for something they do not like to eat, just by thinking that it is good for their health. This will only cause them to waste the food. In order to remedy this situation, make a list of foods that you absolutely dislike and do not wish to include in your meals. At the same time, list out foods that you do like and aim at preparing them in a healthy way. For example, if you dislike kale then substitute it with spinach. If you like potatoes then prep them to make mashed potatoes instead of fries.

Giving up

Many people end up giving up on the activity thinking they are incapable of keeping up with doing it. But it is important to understand that everything takes a little time to settle down. You cannot expect to see overnight results. You have to remain patient and ensure that you do not give up on it just because it isn't giving you desired results. Have an end goal in mind and work towards the same. For example, if you plan to lose 20 pounds in a year then make a different meal plan at the beginning of each month and keep going until the year is up. Giving up half way will not only impact your confidence in a negative manner but also undo some of the positive effects of the activity.

Chapter 5: Basic Meal Prepping Tips

Here are a few basic meal-prepping tips to follow.

➢ It is important to freeze all those foods that you will not be consuming in three days. This is done to maintain the flavor and nutrition of the meals. You must also ensure that they remain fresh and do not spoil. It will be ideal to pack such meals in Ziploc bags or cling film so that there is always room for more. Adding them to containers is also an option, but they can take up more space in the freezer.

➢ Remember that you cannot leave the food in the freezer for too long. In fact, some foods cannot even be kept in the freezer. You have to refer to a guide provided by the FDA that clearly mentions what can be kept in the freezer and what cannot. It is ideal not to freeze carbs, as they can turn soggy.

➢ You can thaw the ingredients by placing them in the fridge the night before, as it will be easier for you to cook with them. But in case you do not have the time to do so or forgot to do so, then an Instant Pot can come in handy. You do not have to worry about thawing it and can simply add it to the pot to cook. You can thaw meats, vegetables and other such ingredients.

➢ You can use your calorie intake as a guide to prepare the meals as that way you will know exactly how much needs to be prepared. On an average, a man will require about 2500 calories while a woman will require 2000 calories. But this can vary depending on the age and other factors. You can speak to a nutritionist to know how many calories you need to consume and prep the meals accordingly.

➢ Avoid adding hot elements to containers and placing them in the fridge. This can modify the flavor and nutritional value of the food. Allow the prepared meals to completely cool down before adding them to the container and storing them.

➢ You can use canning and dehydration techniques to store foods for longer. This is especially useful to store those vegetables that are seasonal. For example, you can pressure can turnips when they are in season. Canning is a technique where you add the chopped vegetables to sterilized jars and top it with hot water. You then close the lid tightly in order to create an internal pressure.

➢ Dehydration involves doing away with the moisture content in the foods. You can use a dehydrator for the same or simply sun-dry the ingredients. Sun drying can take some time but is a cheaper technique to adopt. A dehydrator will do the job faster. Once done, you can add it to Ziploc bags and store in the fridge or freezer. You can add the dehydrated food to warm water and rehydrate them.

Chapter 6: Meal Prep Breakfast Recipes

Anti-inflammatory Turmeric Smoothie with Pineapple & Blueberries

Serves: 2

Ingredients:

- 3 cups pineapple chunks
- 2 cups kale or spinach, discard hard stems and ribs, torn
- ½ teaspoon ground turmeric
- 2 tablespoons chia seeds
- A large pinch pepper powder
- 2 ½ cups almond milk

Method:

1. Place the pineapple chunks on a baking sheet and freeze. Freeze the greens that you are using.
2. Divide and transfer the frozen pineapple and greens into 2 freezer safe jars or zip lock bags (1 serve per jar)
3. Add the rest of the ingredients except milk. Close the lid or seal the bag.
4. Place in the freezer until use.
5. To use: Remove from the freezer and thaw for a while.
6. Empty the jars into a blender. Add milk. Blend until smooth.
7. Pour into glasses and serve.

Blueberry Coconut Water Smoothie (with Hemp Hearts)

Serves: 2

Ingredients:

- 3 cups blueberries
- 1 cup low fat yogurt
- 2 tablespoons hemp hearts
- 2 cups coconut water
- ½ teaspoon coconut extract

Method:

1. Place the berries on a baking sheet and freeze.
2. Divide and transfer the frozen berries into freezer safe jars or zip lock bags (1 serve per jar).
3. Add hemp hearts and coconut extract. Close the lid or seal the bag.
4. Place in the freezer until use.
5. To use: Remove from the freezer and thaw for a while.
6. Empty the jars into a blender. Add yogurt and coconut water. Blend until smooth.
7. Pour into glasses and serve.

Green Mango Super Food Smoothie

Serves: 2

Ingredients:

- 2 cups spinach
- 3 cups mango chunks
- 2 tablespoons chia seeds
- 2 ½ cups almond milk
- 2 teaspoons ground flax
- ¼ teaspoon almond extract

Method:

1. Place the mango chunks on a baking sheet and freeze. Freeze the spinach.
2. Divide and transfer the frozen mango and greens into 2 freezer safe jars or zip lock bags (1 serve per jar)
3. Add rest of the ingredients except milk. Close the lid or seal the bag.
4. Place in the freezer until use.
5. To use: Remove from the freezer and thaw for a while.
6. Empty the jars into a blender. Add milk. Blend until smooth.
7. Pour into glasses and serve.

Goji Peach Cherry Smoothie

Serves: 2

Ingredients:

- 2 cups cherries, pitted
- 2 tablespoons goji berries
- 1 cup peach slices
- 2 ½ cups almond milk
- 2 teaspoons ground flax
- 2 tablespoons chia seeds
- 2 cups kale or spinach, discard hard stems and ribs (optional)

Method:

1. Place the fruits on a baking sheet and freeze. Freeze the greens that you are using.
2. Divide and transfer the frozen fruits and greens into 2 freezer safe jars or zip lock bags (1 serve per jar)
3. Add rest of the ingredients except milk. Close the lid or seal the bag.
4. Place in the freezer until use.
5. To use: Remove from the freezer and thaw for a while.
6. Empty the jars into a blender. Add milk. Blend until smooth.
7. Pour into glasses and serve.

Note: Goji berries are not to be used by pregnant women.

Strawberry Mango Chai Smoothie

Serves: 2

Ingredients:

- 2 cups spinach
- 1 ½ cups strawberries, sliced
- 1 ½ cups mango chunks
- 2 scoops vanilla or strawberry protein powder
- 2 ½ cups almond milk
- 2 teaspoons ground flax
- ¼ teaspoon vanilla extract
- ¼ teaspoon chai spiced blend

Method:

1. Place the fruits on a baking sheet and freeze. Freeze the spinach.
2. Divide and transfer the frozen fruits and spinach into 2 freezer safe jars or zip lock bags (1 serve per jar).
3. Add rest of the ingredients except milk. Close the lid or seal the bag.
4. Place in the freezer until use.
5. To use: Remove from the freezer and thaw for a while.
6. Empty the jars into a blender. Add milk. Blend until smooth.
7. Pour into glasses and serve.

Orange Creamsicle Protein Smoothie

Serves: 2

Ingredients:

- 4 scoops vanilla protein powder
- 1 banana, sliced
- 2 teaspoons orange zest (optional)
- 1 cup water
- 1 cup almond milk
- 6 ounces orange juice concentrate
- 2 teaspoons honey

Method:

1. Place the bananas on a baking sheet and freeze.
2. Divide and transfer the frozen bananas into freezer safe jars or zip lock bags (1 serve per jar).
3. Add rest of the ingredients except milk and water. Close the lid or seal the bag.
4. Place in the freezer until use.
5. To use: Remove from the freezer and thaw for a while.
6. Empty the jars into a blender. Add milk and water. Blend until smooth.
7. Pour into glasses and serve.

Protein Frosty Shake

Serves: 2

Ingredients:

- 4 scoops chocolate protein powder
- 1 banana, sliced
- ½ teaspoon vanilla extract
- 2 cups almond milk
- 1 teaspoon xanthan gum

Method:

1. Place the bananas on a baking sheet and freeze.
2. Divide and transfer the frozen bananas into freezer safe jars or zip lock bags (1 serve per jar).
3. Add rest of the ingredients except milk. Close the lid or seal the bag.
4. Place in the freezer until use.
5. To use: Remove from the freezer and thaw for a while.
6. Empty the jars into a blender. Add milk and water. Blend until smooth.
7. Pour into glasses and serve with crushed ice.

Make Ahead Tofu Scramble & Breakfast Sweet Potatoes

Serves: 3-4

Ingredients:

- ¾ pound sweet potato, peeled, chopped into ½ inch cubes
- 1 teaspoon chili powder
- ½ tablespoon olive oil
- ¼ teaspoon salt or to taste

For tofu scramble:

- 1 small red onion, finely chopped
- ½ block extra firm tofu, crumbled
- 1 cup asparagus, chopped
- 1 bell pepper, finely chopped
- ½ teaspoon ground coriander
- ½ teaspoon ground cumin
- Pepper to taste
- Salt to taste

Method:

1. Place sweet potatoes in a bowl. Add oil, chili powder and salt and toss well. Transfer on to a baking sheet.

2. Bake in a preheated oven at 425 F for 25-30 minutes. Toss the sweet potatoes half way through baking.

3. Meanwhile, place a nonstick pan over medium heat. Add oil. When the oil is heated, add onion, asparagus and bell pepper and sauté for the vegetables are soft.

4. Add rest of the ingredients and sauté for a couple of minutes until well combined.

5. Divide the sweet potatoes into 3-4 containers. Add tofu. Close the lid and store in the refrigerator until use.

6. It can be stored up to 4 days in the refrigerator.

7. To serve: Transfer into a microwave safe dish and microwave on high for a minute.

8. Alternately, add into a pan and heat thoroughly.

Simple Vegan Omelet

Serves: 2

Ingredients:

For omelet:

- 10 ounces firm silken tofu, drained, pat dried
- 4 large cloves garlic, minced
- 4 tablespoons nutritional yeast
- ½ teaspoon paprika
- Pepper to taste
- Salt to taste
- 2 teaspoons cornstarch
- 4 tablespoons hummus
- 1 teaspoon olive oil

For the filling:

- 2 ½ cups vegetables of your choice
- 2 teaspoons olive oil
- Salt to taste
- Pepper to taste

To serve:

- 2-3 tablespoons olive oil
- Salsa as required
- A handful fresh herbs, chopped
- ½ cup vegan parmesan cheese, shredded

Method:

1. For the omelet batter: Place a heatproof skillet over medium heat. Add oil. When the oil is heated, add garlic and sauté until light brown.
2. Remove from heat and add the sautéed garlic into a blender. Add rest of the ingredients of the omelet into the blender and blend until smooth. Add a little water if required and blend again. The batter should not be very thick. So add water accordingly. Transfer into an airtight container and refrigerate until use.
3. For the filling: Place the same skillet back on heat. Add oil. When the oil is heated, add vegetables, salt and pepper and sauté until tender. Remove from heat and set aside in the refrigerator in an airtight container until use.
4. To use: Remove both the containers from the refrigerator 30 minutes before making the omelet.
5. Place a medium size ovenproof nonstick pan over medium heat. Add about tablespoon oil. Swirl the pan so that the oil spreads all over the skillet.
6. When the oil is heated, pour half the omelet batter onto the pan. Swirl the pan so that the batter spreads or spread with the back of a spoon carefully.
7. Cook until the edges are getting to be dry. Remove the pan from heat and place in an oven.
8. Bake in a preheated oven at 375 F for about 10-15 minutes until brown -golden brown (as per your choice). Keep a check on the omelet after about 10 minutes of cooking.
9. Remove from the oven and spread half the vegetables on it. Bake for a couple of minutes. Gently slide a spatula below the omelet to loosen it. Top with a little

salsa, herbs and cheese and fold over. Carefully slide on to a plate and serve.

10. Repeat steps 6-9 to make the other omelet.

Homemade Granola Bars

Serves: 32 bars

Ingredients:

- 4 cups old fashioned rolled oats
- 1 cup shredded coconut, unsweetened
- 2/3 cup honey
- 4 teaspoons vanilla extract
- 1 cup wheat germ, toasted
- 2/3 cup maple syrup
- ½ teaspoon salt
- ½ cup walnuts, chopped into small pieces
- ½ cup almonds, chopped into small pieces
- ½ cup pecans, chopped into small pieces
- ½ cup cashew, chopped into small pieces
- ½ cup dried cranberries, chopped into small pieces
- 1 cup raisins, chopped into small pieces
- ½ cup dried cherries, chopped into small pieces
- ½ cup dried apricots, chopped into small pieces
- ½ cup dried blueberries, chopped into small pieces

Method:

1. Line a large baking dish or 2 smaller baking dishes with parchment paper. Grease it with butter. Set aside.
2. Spread oats and all the nuts on a rimmed baking sheet.

3. Bake in a preheated oven at 300 F for 10 minutes. Stir after 5 minutes of baking. Keep a check on the oven so that you don't end up with burnt stuff.

4. Remove from the oven and transfer into a large bowl. Let it cool for 10 minutes.

5. Add rest of the ingredients and stir until well combined.

6. Transfer the entire contents into the prepared baking dish. Spread it all over the dish with a spatula. Press it down tightly to the bottom of the pan else it will break after baking.

7. Bake in a preheated oven at 300 F for about 25 minutes or until golden brown.

8. Remove from the oven and cool completely.

9. Chop into 32 squares. Place them in an airtight container or in a zip lock container in the freezer until use.

Sweet Potato Kale Hash

Serves: 8

Ingredients:

- 4 tablespoons extra virgin olive oil
- 2 large sweet potatoes, peeled, cubed
- 1 yellow onion, finely chopped
- 2 red bell peppers, finely chopped
- 8 cups kale, discard hard ribs and stems, torn
- 2 tablespoons garlic, minced
- 8 chicken sausages, precooked, sliced
- 4 tablespoons balsamic vinegar
- Salt to taste
- Pepper to taste

Method:

1. Place a skillet over medium heat. Add oil. When the oil is heated, add onions, sweet potatoes, pepper and sausages and sauté until the onions turn translucent.

2. Add kale and sauté until kale wilts. Sprinkle salt, pepper and vinegar. Mix well.

3. Serve if desired. Store the remaining hash in an airtight container in the refrigerator. It can last for 2-3 days.

4. Remove from the oven and heat thoroughly before serving.

Savory Breakfast Muffins

Serves: 24

Ingredients:

- 12 large eggs
- 1 cup cheddar cheese, shredded
- 1 cup red bell pepper, chopped
- ½ cup Canadian bacon, chopped
- ½ cup fresh parsley, chopped
- 2/3 cup old fashioned oats
- 2 cups flour
- 2 tablespoons baking powder
- ½ teaspoon ground cinnamon
- 1 teaspoon salt or to taste
- ½ teaspoon pepper or to taste
- ½ cup applesauce, unsweetened

Method:

1. Whisk together in a bowl, eggs and applesauce until well incorporated.

2. Add all the dry ingredients into a bowl and mix well. Pour the egg mixture into the bowl of dry ingredients and mix until well incorporated.

3. Add cheese, bacon, bell pepper and parsley and stir.

4. Grease 2 muffin pans (12 muffins each) with nonstick cooking spray. Pour the batter into the muffin pans (fill up to 2/3).

5. Place the muffin tins in a preheated oven. Bake at 375 F for 15-20 minutes or until a toothpick when inserted in the center comes out clean.

6. Remove from the oven and place on a wire rack to cool. Loosen the edges with a knife and invert on to a plate.

7. Serve.

8. To store: Wrap each muffin with plastic wrap and place in a freezer bag or airtight container. Place in the freezer until use.

9. To use: remove from the freezer, discard the plastic wrap and wrap it in a paper towel.

10. Microwave on high for 30-45 seconds and serve.

Loaded Breakfast Stuffed Peppers

Serves: 16

Ingredients:

- 8 large bell pepper, halved, deseeded
- 1 cup breakfast cooked potatoes
- 1 cup spinach leaves, chopped
- Salt to taste
- Pepper to taste
- 18 large eggs
- 1 cup cooked quinoa
- 2/3 cup cheese, shredded + extra to top
- 1 cup cooked or canned black beans, drained

Method:

1. Place the bell pepper halves on a baking sheet and bake in a preheated oven at 400 F for 5 minutes. Remove from oven and set aside.

2. Add eggs into a bowl and beat well. Add rest of the ingredients and mix well.

3. Pour the egg mixture into the bell pepper halves. Sprinkle cheese over it.

4. Place the baking sheet back in the oven and bake for about 20 minutes or the eggs are cooked according to the consistency you desire.

5. Serve immediately.

6. Place the unused baked peppers in an airtight container. Refrigerate until use. It can last 4-5 days in the refrigerator.

7. To serve: Heat in an oven or in a microwave and serve.

Bacon n Eggs

Serves 2

Ingredients:

- 4 eggs
- 1 cup spinach, finely shredded
- ½ cup cheese or to taste, shredded + extra to top
- 1 cup bacon, cooked, crumbled
- Salt to taste
- Pepper to taste

Method:

1. Mix together the eggs, spinach, cheese, salt and pepper in a large bowl.
2. Pour into masons jar.
3. Microwave on high for 1 ½ to 2 minutes. Check it in between if it is set.
4. When done, remove from the microwave.
5. Top with bacon and extra cheese if you desire.
6. Tightly screw the lids.
7. Store in the refrigerator until use.
8. To use: Remove the jars from the refrigerator, uncover the jar.
9. Heat in the microwave for 40-50 seconds and serve.

Freezer Breakfast Burritos

Serves: 8

Ingredients:

- 16 large eggs
- 2 tablespoons extra virgin olive oil
- 2 red peppers, finely minced
- 2 tablespoons garlic, minced
- 1 red onion, finely minced
- 8 pieces thick cut bacon, cooked until crisp
- 8 multigrain or whole wheat tortillas
- Salt to taste
- Pepper to taste
- 2-3 tablespoons milk

Method:

1. Whisk together eggs and milk in a bowl.

2. Place a saucepan over medium heat. Add oil. When the oil is heated, add garlic and sauté until fragrant.

3. Add onion and red pepper and sauté until onions are translucent. Pour the egg mixture and sauté until it is cooked. Remove from heat.

4. Place the tortillas on your work area. Divide the egg mixture between the tortillas. Place a piece of bacon over it. Sprinkle cheese. Wrap tightly.

5. Wrap the burrito first in wax paper and then in foil. Place in the freezer. It can last for 1 month in the freezer.

6. To use: Unwrap the burrito and place on a microwave safe plate. Microwave for 2-3 minutes. Turn the burrito once half way through heating.

7. Remove from the microwave and serve after a minute.

Yogurt and Granola Parfait

Serves 3

Ingredients:

- 2 cups plain, low fat yogurt
- 2 cups fruits or berries of your choice
- ¼ cup honey
- ¾ cup rolled oats
- ¼ cup nuts, chopped and seeds of your choice
- ½ tablespoon olive oil
- ½ teaspoon cinnamon
- ¼ teaspoon vanilla extract
- A pinch of salt

Method:

1. Grease a baking dish with cooking spray or butter and set aside.
2. Mix together the oats, nuts, oil, cinnamon, vanilla, salt and 2 tablespoons honey. Mix until well coated.
3. Spread evenly on a greased baking dish.
4. Bake for around 45 minutes, stirring it every 15 minutes.
5. The granola should be golden brown in color when it is ready. Otherwise bake for another 10-15 minutes or until done.
6. Take 3 masons jars. Divide and spoon yogurt in it, divide and pour the remaining honey over it.

7. Next layer it with half the fruits and followed by half the granola.

8. Repeat the above layer.

9. Tightly screw on the lids and refrigerate.

10. It can store up to 3 days.

11. Serve either cold or at room temperature.

Chocolate Peanut Butter Protein Baked Oatmeal Cups

Serves: 24

Ingredients:

- 4 tablespoons chia seeds mixed with ¾ cup water or 4 large eggs
- 2 cups cashew milk or almond milk, unsweetened
- ½ cup pure maple syrup or 30 drops liquid stevia
- 6 cup old fashioned oats
- 2 scoops chocolate protein powder
- 6 medium to large very ripe bananas, mashed
- ½ cup creamy peanut butter
- 1 teaspoon vanilla extract
- 4 tablespoons cocoa powder
- A large pinch salt
- 2 tablespoons baking powder

Method:

1. Add milk, peanut butter, maple syrup or stevia and vanilla into a bowl and mix well.

2. Add chia seed mixture or eggs and mix well.

3. Add rest of the ingredients into a bowl and add into the above mixture.

4. Pour it in muffin tins up to ¾; make sure the tins are greased.

5. Bake in a preheated oven at 350 F for about 20-25 minutes or until a toothpick when inserted in the center comes out clean.

6. Cool on a wire rack. Remove from the molds and store in an airtight container.

7. Store in the refrigerator. It can last for 5-6 days in the refrigerator.

Chapter 7: Meal Prep Snack Recipes

Banana Sandwiches

Serves: 4-8

Ingredients:

- 2 bananas, peeled, sliced into 1 cm thick slices
- Peanut butter (sweet and salty) as required

Method:

1. Spread butter on half the banana slices. Cover with the other half and refrigerate until use.
2. It can last for a day.

Grapes on a Stick

Serves: 8

Ingredients:

- 32 large grapes

Method:

1. Stick a toothpick in each of the grapes.
2. Freeze and serve later.

Pistachio Date Bites

Serves 12

Ingredients:

- 24 soft dates, pitted
- 3 tablespoons almond butter
- 1/3 cup pistachio nuts crushed
- 2 tablespoons oil

Method:

1. Blend together dates and almond butter in a blender until smooth.
2. Transfer into a bowl. Grease your hands with a little oil.
3. Form small balls of the mixture.
4. Place the crushed pistachio in a plate. Dredge the balls in the pistachio. Coat well.
5. Place in an airtight container and refrigerate until use.
6. It can last for a week in the refrigerator

Kale Chips

Serves: 4

Ingredients:

- 1 bunch of kale leaves, discard hard ribs and stems
- Cooking spray
- Salt to taste
- Chili powder to taste

Method:

1. Rinse and drain the kale leaves. Pat the leaves dry with a kitchen towel. Tear the leaves.

2. Spray the leaves with cooking spray. Sprinkle salt and chili powder over it. Keep aside for a while.

3. Spread the leaves on a baking sheet on a baking sheet in a single layer. Do not overlap. Bake in batches if required

4. Bake in a preheated oven at 250 degree F until crisp.

5. When cooled, store in an airtight container until use. It can last for 3-4 days.

Mixed treat

Serves: 12

Ingredients:

- 1 cup mixed nuts of your choice, chopped
- 1 cup seeds of your choice, toasted if desired
- 1 cup dried fruits of your choice, chopped

Method:

1. Mix together all the ingredients in a bowl.
2. Take small zip lock pouches. Add about ¼ cup of the mixture in it. Seal and store until use.

Baked Oatmeal Cups with Berries and Bananas

Serves: 24 -30

Ingredients:

- 4 large eggs, lightly beaten
- 2 almond milk, unsweetened
- 2 tablespoons honey
- 5 cups old fashioned oats
- 4 large very ripe bananas, mashed
- 2 teaspoons vanilla extract
- 2 tablespoons cinnamon powder
- 4 cups fresh blueberries or raspberries
- 3 teaspoons baking powder
- Cooking spray

Method:

1. Add bananas, honey and eggs into a bowl and mix well.

2. Add rest of the ingredients into a bowl and add into the above mixture.

3. Pour in muffin tins up to ¾; make sure the tins are greased. Sprinkle blueberries over it.

4. Bake in a preheated oven at 350 F for about 20-25 minutes, until golden brown.

5. Cool on a wire rack. Remove from the molds and store in an airtight container.

6. Store in the refrigerator. It can last for 5-6 days in the refrigerator.

Sweet potato Chips

Serves: 8

Ingredients:

- 2 large sweet potatoes, peeled, cut into thin round slices like chips
- Cooking spray
- Salt to taste
- Seasoning of your choice
- Pepper to taste

Method:

1. Sprinkle salt, pepper and seasoning on the sweet potato slices. Spray with cooking spray.

2. Spread the leaves on a baking sheet on a baking sheet in a single layer. Do not overlap. Bake in batches if required.

3. Bake in a preheated oven at 250 degree F until crisp.

4. When cooled, store in an airtight container until use. It can last for 6-7 days.

Ham, Swiss, and Spinach Roll Ups

Serves: 4

Ingredients:

- 4 slices uncured deli ham
- 2 slices Swiss cheese, halved
- 4 tablespoons hummus
- 8 baby spinach leaves

Method:

1. Place the ham slices on your work area. Spread about a tablespoon of hummus over it. Place half slice of cheese and spinach leaves on top. Roll tightly and place with its seam side down.

2. Serve later. It can store for 2 days if refrigerated.

Beef and Cheddar "No Bread" Roll Ups

Serves: 4

Ingredients:

- 4 slices thinly sliced roast beef
- Thousand Island yogurt dressing as required
- 1 tomato, chopped
- 1 onion, chopped

Method:

1. Place the beef slices on your work area. Spread dressing over it. Place cheese, onions and tomatoes over it. Roll tightly and place with its seam side down.

2. Serve later. It can store for 1 day if refrigerated.

Veggie Snack Packs

Serves: 6

Ingredients:

- 1 cup mixed bell peppers, thinly sliced like matchsticks
- 1 cup carrots, thinly sliced like matchsticks
- 1 cup cucumber, thinly sliced like matchsticks
- Hummus as required

Method:

1. Mix together all the vegetables in a bowl and place in the refrigerator.
2. Serve with hummus.
3. The vegetables can last 2-3 days in the refrigerator.

Cottage Cheese-Filled Avocado

Serves: 8

Ingredients:

- 4 avocadoes, peeled, pitted, halved lengthwise
- 8 ounces 1% cottage cheese, crumbled

Method:

1. Fill the avocadoes with cottage and refrigerate until use.
2. It can last for 2 days. Season with salt and pepper if desired.

Warm Pear with Cinnamon Ricotta

Serves: 4

Ingredients:

- 4 small pears, halved, cored
- 1 teaspoon ground cinnamon
- 1 cup part skim ricotta cheese

Method:

1. Place the pears on a baking sheet and broil in an oven for 10-12 minutes until tender

2. Mix together cinnamon and ricotta in a bowl. Top this mixture over the pears.

3. Refrigerate until use. It can last for 2 days.

Roasted Edamame

Serves: 4

Ingredients:

- 4 cups edamame
- 1 tablespoon olive oil
- Salt to taste
- Pepper to taste

Method:

1. Mix together all the ingredients into a bowl. Transfer on to a baking sheet.

2. Bake in a preheated oven at 300 F for about an hour.

3. Cool and serve later. It can last for 2-3 days in the refrigerator.

Chapter 8: Meal Recipes

Chicken Curry with Spinach

Serves: 4

Ingredients:

- 2 chicken breasts, boneless, skinless, chopped into bite sized pieces
- 1 small onion, halved, sliced
- 1 cup chicken stock
- 1 small red bell pepper, thinly sliced
- 3 bunches fresh spinach, rinsed
- ½ tablespoons fresh ginger, minced
- 2 cloves garlic, sliced
- 1 teaspoon curry powder
- ¼ teaspoon turmeric powder
- 6 tablespoons coconut milk
- White pepper powder to taste
- Salt to taste

Method:

1. Boil a pot of water and add spinach to it. Boil for a minute and drain. Press to squeeze out the excess moisture. Sprinkle salt and pepper and set aside.
2. Place a nonstick pan over medium low heat. Add onions and sauté for 5 minutes.

3. Add ginger and garlic and sauté for a couple of minutes until fragrant.

4. Add turmeric and curry powder and sauté for a few seconds.

5. Add stock, chicken, coconut milk and simmer for 5-6 minutes. Add bell pepper and cook until the chicken is tender.

6. To serve: Place blanched spinach on serving plates and place chicken mixture over it.

Tomato Fennel Gratin

Serves: 4

Ingredients:

- 10 small Roma tomatoes, slice into ¼ inch thick rounds
- 4 ounces crème fraiche
- 2 large or 4 small fennel bulbs, discard stalks, halved, thinly sliced, steamed
- 1 cup parmesan, finely grated
- 4 tablespoons black olive tapenade
- Salt to taste
- Freshly ground black pepper to taste
- A handful fresh thyme leaves, chopped

Method:

1. Add steamed fennel, crème fraiche, tapenade, half the thyme leaves, salt, pepper and Parmesan into a bowl. Transfer into a greased baking dish.

2. Place the tomato slices over the fennel layer. Overlap the tomatoes while placing it.

3. Sprinkle salt and pepper. Sprinkle cheese and remaining thyme leaves.

4. Bake in a preheated oven 425° F for about 20 minutes or until light brown in color. Let it sit in the oven for 5 minutes.

5. Serve.

Potato Rounds with Fresh Lemon

Serves: 6

Ingredients:

- 1 ½ pounds fingerling potatoes, scrubbed, sliced into 1/8 inch thick rounds
- 3 teaspoons dried oregano
- 1 ½ tablespoons extra virgin olive oil, divided
- 3 teaspoons lemon zest, grated
- Coarsely ground black pepper to taste
- Salt to taste

Method:

1. Add potatoes, pepper, oregano and half the oil into a bowl and toss well.

2. Transfer on to a greased baking sheet and spread it in a single layer. Bake in batches if necessary.

3. Bake in a preheated oven 450° F for about 20 minutes or until golden brown in color. It should be tender inside and crisp outside. Turn the potatoes half way through baking.

4. When done, remove from the oven. Sprinkle remaining oil, lemon zest and salt and toss well. Serve immediately.

Kale Chickpea Mash

Serves: 4

Ingredients:

- 4 cups cooked chickpeas
- 4 tablespoons garlic, minced
- 2 bunches kale, discard hard ribs and stems, chopped
- 2 shallots, chopped
- 4 tablespoons extra virgin olive oil
- 4 tablespoons liquid aminos or soy sauce
- Salt to taste
- 1 teaspoon dried thyme

Method:

1. Place a skillet over medium heat. Add oil. When oil is hot, add onion and garlic. Sauté until onions are golden brown.

2. Add kale and sauté until the kale wilts. Add rest of the ingredients and cook for a while.

3. Mash with a fork to the consistency you desire and serve.

Asian Sautéed Cauliflower

Serves: 4-6

Ingredients:

- 2 medium heads cauliflower, trimmed, cut into big pieces
- 4 tablespoons soy sauce
- 4 tablespoons rice vinegar or lemon juice
- 10 tablespoons vegetable broth
- 4 cloves garlic, pressed
- 1 teaspoon fresh ginger, grated
- 2 tablespoons extra virgin olive oil
- 2 tablespoons honey
- 1 fresh cilantro, chopped
- Salt to taste
- White pepper powder to taste
- 1 tablespoon dry mustard

Method:

1. Place a large skillet or wok over medium heat. Add 2 tablespoons broth and cauliflower, cover and cook for 5 minutes.

2. Mix together rest of the ingredients and add to cauliflower. Mix well and remove from heat.

3. Cover and set aside for a few minutes before serving.

Shepherd's Pie

Serves: 4

Ingredients:

- 1 pound ground beef
- 2 cloves garlic, minced
- 1 medium yellow onion, chopped
- 1 carrot, peeled, chopped
- 4 ounce mushrooms, sliced
- ½ bag frozen peas, thawed
- ½ can tomato paste
- 1 tablespoon balsamic vinegar
- ½ tablespoon fresh rosemary, chopped
- 1 teaspoon fresh thyme, chopped
- 2-3 medium sized sweet potatoes
- ¼ cup light coconut milk or low fat milk
- 1 ½ tablespoons butter
- Sea salt to taste
- Pepper powder to taste

Method:

1. Bake the sweet potatoes in a preheated oven at 350° F until soft. Cool.

2. When cooled, peel the sweet potatoes and mash with a potato masher. Place the mashed sweet potatoes in a

bowl. Add milk, 1-tablespoon butter, sea salt and pepper. Mash well and set aside.

3. In a large skillet add ½ tablespoon butter. Keep on medium heat. Add garlic and meat. Sauté.

4. Cook until the meat is browned and keep aside.

5. To the same skillet add onions, carrots and mushrooms and sauté until the onions are pink and carrots are soft.

6. Toss the meat in the pan. Add salt, balsamic vinegar, tomato paste, rosemary and thyme.

7. Cook until the liquid is dried up.

8. Add peas. Mix well. Transfer this mixture into a large baking dish.

9. Spread the mashed sweet potato mixture over the meat mixture.

10. Place the baking dish into a preheated oven at 350° F and bake for 15-20 minutes or longer if you want it browner.

Hot Paprika Chicken Breast

Serves: 6

Ingredients:

- 6 chicken breasts, skinless, boneless, chop into chunks
- 4 tablespoons olive oil
- 4 tablespoons Spanish smoked paprika
- 3 tablespoons lemon juice
- 1 ½ tablespoons maple syrup
- 3 teaspoons garlic, minced
- Salt to taste
- Pepper powder to taste

Method:

1. Mix together all the ingredients except the chicken to make the sauce.
2. Season the chicken with salt and pepper.
3. Pour 1/3 of the sauce to a casserole dish. Place the chicken pieces on top of it.
4. Pour the remaining sauce all over the chicken pieces.
5. Bake in a preheated oven at 350° F for about 30 minutes or until done.

Seared Salmon

Serves: 6

Ingredients:

- 2 ½ pounds wild salmon fillet, skinned, cut into big pieces
- ½ cup lemon juice
- 4 teaspoons canola oil
- ½ teaspoon salt, divided
- 3 tablespoons unsalted butter, chopped coarsely
- 2 teaspoons green peppercorns soaked in vinegar

Method:

1. Season salmon pieces with half the salt.
2. Place a large nonstick skillet over medium high heat. Add half the oil.
3. Add half the salmon pieces and cook for 2-3 minutes and flip sides. Cook until the salmon pieces turn opaque in the center.
4. Repeat step 2 and 3 with the remaining salmon pieces.
5. When done add the first batch of seared salmon back to the pan. Stir for a minute and remove from heat.
6. Add lemon juice, peppercorns (rinse and crush them before using), butter, and remaining salt. Then swirl the pan so that butter melts and peppercorn are well blended in the butter.
7. To serve: Place salmon pieces on individual plates and pour sauce over it and serve.

Butternut Squash Sauté

Serves: 3

Ingredients:

- 2 small butternut squash, peeled, deseeded, chopped into ½ inch cubes
- 2 teaspoons ground cumin
- 2 tablespoons olive oil
- 1 teaspoon ground cinnamon
- Freshly ground black pepper to taste
- Salt to taste

Method:

1. Place a skillet over high heat. Add oil. When the oil is heated, add squash and toss well.
2. Add rest of the ingredients and sauté until tender and brown on the outside. Toss frequently.
3. Serve hot.

Homemade Burgers

Serves: 12

Ingredients:

- 2 eggs
- 2 ½ pounds ground beef
- ½ teaspoon dried minced onion
- 2 tablespoons coconut flour
- 1 teaspoon chili powder
- 1 ½ teaspoons garlic powder
- ¼ teaspoon red pepper flakes or to taste
- 1 teaspoon dried oregano
- 1 teaspoon dried basil
- ½ teaspoon ground coriander
- Black pepper to taste
- Salt to taste
- Whole wheat burger buns to serve, as required
- Cooking spray

Method:

1. Mix together all the ingredients except burger buns in a large bowl with your hands. Shape into patties.

2. Place a nonstick pan over medium heat. Spray with cooking spray. Place patties over it and cook on both the sides.

3. Apply mayonnaise or any spread you desire.

4. Place inside the burger and serve.

5. Place the unused, uncooked burger on a baking sheet and freeze.

6. Once frozen, remove from the baking sheet and place in a freezer safe dish and freeze again.

Roasted Mushrooms with Thyme

Serves: 4-6

Ingredients:

- 2 pounds cremini mushrooms
- 15 fresh thyme sprigs
- 4 tablespoons olive oil
- 8 cloves garlic, minced
- 1 tablespoon ghee or coconut oil
- Sea salt to taste
- Freshly ground black pepper to taste

Method:

1. Place an ovenproof skillet over medium heat. Add ghee. When the ghee melts, add garlic and thyme. Sauté for a few seconds until fragrant. Remove from heat.

2. Place the mushrooms in the skillet over the garlic and thyme with the cap side down. Sprinkle salt and pepper.

3. Sprinkle olive oil all over the mushrooms.

4. Bake in a preheated oven at 375° F for about 20-25 minutes.

5. Remove the skillet from the oven. Mix well with the drippings in the skillet and serve.

Sausage and Cauliflower Bake

Serves: 8

Ingredients:

- 1 Large cauliflower, chopped into florets
- 8 pork sausages
- 10 tablespoons coconut cream
- 8 slices low fat cheese or non dairy cheese
- 1 teaspoon salt or to taste
- Pepper powder to taste

Method:

1. Steam the cauliflower florets. Mash with a potato masher.
2. Add coconut cream, salt and pepper.
3. Place a nonstick skillet over medium heat. Add sausages and cook until done.
4. When cool enough to handle, slice the sausages and add to cauliflower mixture and mix well.
5. Now layer as follows:
6. Add half the cauliflower mixture to a greased baking dish.
7. Lay half the cheese slices.
8. Spread the remaining mixture over the cheese slices.
9. Lay the remaining cheese slices over the cauliflower layer.
10. Place the baking dish in a in a preheated oven and bake at 350° F for around 30 minutes.

Coconut Chicken Curry

Serves: 4

Ingredients:

- 1 ½ pounds chicken breast
- 1 cup coconut milk
- 3 tablespoons canola oil
- 1 ½ cups vegetable broth
- 1 ½ tablespoons mild curry powder
- 3 tablespoons basil, chopped
- ½ package frozen haricots verts, cook according to instructions on the package
- Salt to taste

Method:

1. Mix together 1-tablespoon curry powder and 1-½ tablespoons oil and rub it on to the chicken breast.

2. Place an ovenproof skillet over high heat. Add remaining oil. When oil is heated, add the chicken and cook until brown on all the sides.

3. Remove from heat and place the skillet in a preheated oven.

4. Bake at 350° F for about 15 minutes or until a thermometer when inserted in the center of the chicken shows 155° F.

5. Remove the dish from the oven and cool. When cool enough to handle, slice the chicken into thin slices.

6. Pour a little coconut milk and curry powder to a saucepan and blend until smooth.

7. Add rest of the coconut milk and vegetable broth and place the saucepan over medium heat and simmer until the mixture is slightly thick.

8. Add basil and mix. Remove from heat.

9. To serve: Arrange haricots verts over individual serving plates. Place pork slices over it. Pour sauce over pork and serve.

Sausage and Cauliflower Bake

Serves: 8

Ingredients:

- 1 Large cauliflower, chopped into florets
- 8 pork sausages
- 10 tablespoons coconut cream
- 8 slices low fat cheese or non dairy cheese
- 1 teaspoon salt or to taste
- Pepper powder to taste

Method:

1. Steam the cauliflower florets. Mash with a potato masher.
2. Add coconut cream, salt and pepper.
3. Place a nonstick skillet over medium heat. Add sausages and cook until done.
4. When cool enough to handle, slice the sausages and add to cauliflower mixture and mix well.
5. Now layer as follows:
6. Add half the cauliflower mixture to a greased baking dish.
7. Lay half the cheese slices.
8. Spread the remaining mixture over the cheese slices.
9. Lay the remaining cheese slices over the cauliflower layer.
10. Place the baking dish in a in a preheated oven and bake at 350° F for around 30 minutes.

Beef and Broccoli Stir Fry

Serves: 3

Ingredients

- 1 pound beef, top steak, cut into ¼ inch slant slices
- 1 large head broccoli, cut into florets, slice the stalk into thin strips
- 6 cloves garlic, minced
- 2 tablespoons fresh ginger, peeled, minced
- 2 red chili peppers, minced
- 2 teaspoons crushed red pepper flakes
- 2 tablespoons apple cider vinegar
- 4 tablespoons canola oil
- 4 tablespoons tamari or coconut aminos or soy sauce
- 3 cups beef broth
- 2 tablespoons sesame seeds
- ¼ cup water

Method:

1. Mix together in a bowl, beef, soy sauce and garlic and marinate for 15-20 minutes.
2. Mix together in a small bowl, broth, vinegar, red pepper flakes and ginger root.
3. Place a large nonstick skillet over medium high heat. Add 2 tablespoons oil. When oil is heated, add only the beef and cook until brown. Remove from the pan and set aside.

4. Place the pan back on heat. Add remaining oil. When oil is heated, add broccoli and chili pepper and sauté for a minute.

5. Add water, cover and cook until broccoli is tender. Stir frequently.

6. Add broth mixture and cooked beef. Simmer for 3-4 minutes.

7. Remove from heat. Sprinkle sesame seeds and serve.

Green, Red and Yellow Rice

Serves: 4

Ingredients:

- 2 cups brown rice, rinsed, cook according to the instructions on the package
- 2 cups green onions, chopped
- ¼ cup garlic, finely chopped
- 2 cups red bell pepper, chopped
- 2 cups frozen corn, thawed
- 2 tablespoons olive oil
- 1 cup fresh cilantro, chopped
- Salt to taste
- Pepper to taste
- Cayenne pepper to taste

Method:

1. Place a large skillet over medium heat. Add oil. When the oil is heated, add garlic and sauté until fragrant. Do not burn it.

2. Add rest of the ingredients except rice and cilantro and sauté for 2-3 minutes.

3. Add rice and cilantro. Mix well and heat thoroughly.

Simply Tasty Black Beans

Serves: 5

Ingredients:

- 1 cup dried black beans, soaked in water overnight, drained, rinsed
- ½ cup onions, chopped
- 1 tablespoon garlic, chopped
- ¼ cup celery, chopped
- 1 cup tomatoes, chopped
- ¼ teaspoon ground cumin
- ½ teaspoon cayenne pepper
- ½ tablespoon honey
- ¼ teaspoon ground cinnamon
- Salt to taste
- Pepper to taste
- 2 sprigs fresh thyme

Method:

1. Place a large saucepan over medium heat. Add oil. When the oil is heated, add onions, garlic and celery and sauté until onions are translucent.

2. Add tomatoes and sauté for a couple of minutes. Add cumin, cinnamon and cayenne pepper. Sauté for a few seconds until fragrant.

3. Add black beans, thyme, honey and enough water to cover the ingredients.

4. Cover and simmer until the beans are tender. If the beans are not cooked and you find there is no liquid in the saucepan, then add some hot water. The beans may take about 1-1 ½ hours to cook.

5. Add salt and pepper and cook for another 10 minutes. Discard the thyme sprigs.

6. Serve hot.

Chicken Taco Pizza

Serves: 8

Ingredients:

- 2 whole wheat pizza crusts, freshly made or frozen
- 2 frozen chicken breasts, skinless, boneless, thawed, chopped into bite sized pieces
- 2 cups frozen corn, thawed
- 2 cups cooked black beans, rinsed, drained
- 1 cup salsa + extra to serve
- 2 cups part skim mozzarella cheese, grated, divided
- ½ cup fresh cilantro, chopped

Method:

1. Lay the pizza crusts on a large baking sheet. Divide salsa and spread over both the crusts. Sprinkle half the cheese over the salsa.

2. Sprinkle beans, corn, and chicken over the cheese. Finally top with the remaining cheese.

3. Bake in a preheated oven 425° F until the cheese is melted and slightly brown.

4. Remove from the oven and sprinkle cilantro on it. Cut into wedges and serve with some salsa.

Pulled Pork Poblano

Serves: 4

Ingredients:

- 1 ½ pounds pork shoulder, trimmed of fat, chopped into 2 inch chunks
- ½ pound tomatillos, husked, quartered
- 1 Serrano pepper, halved, sliced
- 1 poblano pepper or more if you like it hot, deseeded, halved, sliced
- 1 small onion, chopped
- 1 teaspoon safflower oil
- Pepper to taste
- Salt to taste
- 3 cloves garlic, smashed
- ½ teaspoon ground coriander
- 1 ½ teaspoons ground cumin
- Juice of ½ lime
- 2 cups chicken broth

Method:

1. Place a heavy bottomed heatproof pot or Dutch oven over high heat. Add oil. When the oil is heated, add pork and sprinkle salt and pepper over it. Cook until brown.

2. Remove pork with a slotted spoon and set aside. Discard the fat that is remaining in the pot.

3. Place the pot back on heat. Add tomatillos, onion, garlic and peppers and sauté until brown.

4. Add spices, salt and pepper and sauté for a few seconds until fragrant. Add broth and the pork along with the released juices into the pot. Add more broth if required. The pork should be covered with broth.

5. Bring to the boil.

6. Lower heat and cover. Simmer until the pork is tender. It may take 1 ½ - 2 hours.

7. Remove the pork with a slotted spoon and place on your work area. When cool enough to handle, shred with a pair of forks.

8. Meanwhile, remove any fat that is floating on the top. Simmer the liquid until thick. Add lime juice, salt and pepper if necessary.

9. Add the pork back into the pot. Heat thoroughly and serve.

Beef Taco Stuffed Avocadoes

Serves: 5

Ingredients:

- ½ pound ground beef
- ¼ cup onions, finely chopped
- ¼ cup bell pepper, finely chopped
- 2 green onions, thinly sliced
- 1 tablespoon olive oil
- ¼ cup sharp cheddar cheese, grated
- 5 small avocadoes, halved, pitted
- 2 teaspoons taco seasoning or more to taste
- Salt to taste

Method:

1. Place a skillet over medium heat. Add oil. When the oil is heated, add onion and bell pepper and sauté until onions are translucent.

2. Add beef and sauté until beef is nearly cooked. Add taco seasoning and salt and cook for 2-3 minutes.

3. Remove from heat and add cheese. Mix well.

4. Divide and fill the avocadoes with this mixture. Sprinkle green onions on top.

5. Serve immediately.

Creamy Butternut Squash Risotto

Serves: 6

Ingredients:

- 2 cups raw cashews, soaked in water overnight, drained
- 5 cups butternut squash, peeled, deseeded, chopped
- 1 cup onion, chopped
- 6 cloves garlic, minced
- ½ cup fresh parsley, finely chopped
- 3 cups non-dairy milk like soy milk or almond milk
- 1 teaspoon fine sea salt
- 1 teaspoon ground cinnamon
- 2 packages (20 ounce each) frozen brown rice
- 1 ½ cups low sodium vegetable broth or more if required
- 4 tablespoons fresh sage, minced
- ½ teaspoon freshly ground black pepper
- Cooking spray

Method:

1. Place a large pot over medium heat. Add squash and cook until tender. Remove about 1-½ cups of the squash and keep it aside.

2. Let the rest of the squash cook for another 10 minutes or until very soft. Drain and set aside.

3. Meanwhile, blend together in a blender, cashew, softened squash, milk, cinnamon, and salt until smooth and creamy. Set it aside.

4. Place a large skillet over medium heat. Spray with cooking spray. Add onions and garlic and sauté until light brown.

5. Add the cup of squash that was kept aside, brown rice and broth. Cook for 2-3 minutes stirring frequently. If you find it too dry, add some more broth.

6. Add creamy cashew mixture, sage and parsley. Stir and lower heat. Simmer until risotto of the desired thickness is achieved.

7. Remove from heat. Sprinkle black pepper powder and stir. Serve hot.

Coconut Shrimp and Avocadoes

Serves: 2

Ingredients:

- 1 avocado, peeled, pitted, chop into bite sized cubes
- 2 cups shrimp
- 2 teaspoons Sriracha sauce or any other hot sauce
- 1 tablespoon natural peanut butter
- 2 teaspoons shredded coconut
- 2 tablespoons light coconut milk
- Salt to taste
- Cooking spray

Method:

1. Place a nonstick pan over medium heat. Spray with cooking spray.
2. Add coconut milk, peanut butter, salt and hot sauce. Stir until well combined.
3. Add shrimp and cook until shrimp are tender.
4. Remove from heat and sprinkle coconut over it.
5. Place avocadoes on a serving plate. Place the shrimp over it and serve.

Lamb Roast with Veggies

Serves: 2

Ingredients:

- ½ pound lamb stew meat, cut into large cubes
- 2 medium tomatoes
- 1 onion, roughly chopped
- 2 cloves garlic, pressed
- 1 cup button mushrooms, halved
- 2 carrots, peeled, chopped
- 1 tablespoon fresh thyme, finely chopped
- 1 tablespoon fresh rosemary, finely chopped
- 1 cup chicken or lamb stock
- Freshly ground black pepper to taste

Method:

1. Blanch the tomatoes in boiling water until the skin just starts to crack.
2. Strain the tomatoes and place in cold water and peel the skin. Chop the tomatoes into chunks.
3. Add tomatoes to a large baking dish. Add mushrooms, carrots, onions, lamb, salt, pepper, rosemary, thyme and garlic. Mix well.
4. Place the baking dish in a preheated oven at 325° F and bake for about 2 hours or until the lamb is cooked. Stir a couple of times in between.
5. Serve hot.

Power Meatballs

Serves: 5-6

Ingredients:

- 2 pounds lean ground turkey
- 3 teaspoons garlic powder
- 2 teaspoons onion powder
- 2 teaspoons dried basil
- 1 teaspoon red pepper flakes
- 2 teaspoons dried oregano
- 2 eggs
- 1 cup rolled oats
- Salt to taste

Method:

1. Mix together all the ingredients into a bowl using your hands.
2. Form balls of about 1 inch diameter and place on a lined baking sheet
3. Place the baking sheet in a preheated oven at 400° F and bake for about 23-25 minutes.

Easy Tuna Sliders

Serves: 4

Ingredients:

- 2 cans wild albacore tuna
- 2 large cucumbers
- 4 tablespoons spicy mustard
- 2 tablespoons apple cider vinegar
- Salt to taste
- Pepper to taste

Method:

1. Cut the cucumber into around 1/3-inch slices. Drizzle apple cider vinegar on the cucumber and set aside for a while.

2. Mix together tuna and mustard in a bowl.

3. Place cucumber slices on a serving platter. Top each slice with the tuna mixture.

4. Season with salt and pepper and serve

Vegan Mushroom Alfredo

Serves: 8

Ingredients:

- 16 ounces whole wheat spelt rotini or any other whole wheat pasta, cook according to instructions on the package
- 1 pound mixed mushrooms, trimmed, sliced
- 4 tablespoons extra virgin olive oil
- 8 cloves garlic, minced
- 1 cup almonds, sliced, divided
- 1 ½ cups almond milk, unsweetened
- 1 ½ teaspoons fine sea salt, divided
- 1 teaspoon freshly ground black pepper powder
- 4 tablespoons nutritional yeast
- ¼ cup fresh parsley, chopped

Method:

1. Place a large deep skillet or wok over medium high heat. Add oil. When oil is heated, add mushrooms and about a teaspoon salt. Sauté until brown.

2. Add garlic and sauté until fragrant.

3. Meanwhile toast half the almonds and set aside. Add the remaining almonds to a blender and blend along with nutritional yeast and almond milk until smooth and creamy. Add this to the skillet.

4. Add pasta, salt and pepper and toss well.

5. Garnish with toasted almonds and parsley and serve.

Zucchini Pasta Bolognese

Serves: 6

Ingredients:

- 5 whole zucchinis
- 1 can tomato paste
- 2 cans (14.5 ounces each) diced tomatoes
- 2 large yellow onions, grated
- 6 cloves garlic, crushed
- 2 pounds ground lamb
- 2 cups beef broth or chicken broth
- 1/3 cup coconut milk
- 2 cups red wine
- 2 tablespoons coconut aminos or tamari
- 2 tablespoons dried oregano
- ½ cup fresh basil leaves, chopped
- Salt to taste
- Pepper powder to taste
- 2 tablespoons olive oil or coconut oil

Method:

1. Make noodles of zucchinis by using a spiralizer or a julienne peeler and set aside.
2. Place a large saucepan over medium heat. Add oil. When oil is heated, add grated onions.

3. Sauté for a while. Add salt, pepper, and dried oregano and sauté for a couple of minutes.

4. Add garlic and sauté for a couple of minutes until fragrant. Add ground lamb and stir constantly. When beef is light brown, push the lamb all around the pan making space at the center.

5. Add tomato paste in the center and fry for a couple of minutes and slowly mix it in the beef. Add red wine and mix well. Let it cook for a while until the wine almost dries up.

6. Add tomatoes, stock and coconut aminos. Add coconut milk, stir and simmer for 5 minutes.

7. Add basil, stir and simmer for 2-3 minutes.

8. Place the zucchini noodles over individual serving plates. Pour sauce over the noodles and serve. If you don't like the zucchini noodles raw, then sauté in oil for 2-3 minutes.

Chicken Parmesan

Serves: 2

Ingredients:

- 2 chicken breasts, skinless, trimmed
- 2 tablespoons arrowroot flour
- ½ cup almond flour
- 2 eggs, beaten
- ¼ teaspoon onion powder
- ½ teaspoon oregano
- ¼ teaspoon garlic powder
- ½ teaspoon basil
- Salt to taste
- Pepper to taste
- Crushed red pepper flakes to taste

Method:

1. Add flours, spices herbs and salt into a bowl. Mix well.
2. First dip a chicken breast into the egg. Shake off excess egg. Next dredge the chicken into the flour mixture. Dip again into the egg and dredge in the flour. Place on a lined baking sheet.
3. Repeat the above step with the other chicken breast.
4. Bake in a preheated oven at 375° F for about 40 minutes.
5. Top with spaghetti sauce and brown rice noodles or zucchini noodles and serve.

Roast Turkey Breast with Chipotle Chili Sauce

Serves: 8

Ingredients:

- 1 turkey breast, roasted, sliced

For sauce:

- 6 cloves garlic, minced
- 1 large onion, minced
- 4 canned chipotle chilies, minced
- 2 cups chicken broth
- 4 tablespoons tomato paste
- 2 tablespoons fresh oregano, chopped
- 4 tablespoons Dijon mustard
- 4 tablespoons blackstrap molasses
- 1 tablespoon olive oil
- Salt to taste

Method:

1. To make sauce: Place a skillet over medium heat. Add oil. When oil is heated, add onions and sauté until onions are translucent. Add garlic and sauté until fragrant.

2. Add rest of the ingredients and simmer until thickened.

3. Serve roasted turkey with some sauce poured on it.

Shrimp and Bacon with Zoodles

Serves: 8

Ingredients:

- 8 slices uncured bacon, cut into 1 inch pieces
- 2 cups mushrooms, sliced
- 8 ounces smoked salmon, cut into strips
- 8 ounces raw shelled shrimp
- 1 cup coconut cream
- A large pinch Celtic sea salt or to taste
- Freshly ground black pepper to taste

Method:

1. Place a large cast iron skillet over medium heat. Add bacon. Cook until done.
2. Add mushrooms and sauté until tender.
3. Add smoked salmon. Sauté for 2-3 minutes.
4. Add coconut cream and salt. Reduce heat and simmer for a minute.
5. Serve immediately with zucchini noodles.

Sautéed Turkey with Tomatoes and Cilantro

Serves: 6

Ingredients:

- 2 pounds lean ground turkey
- 1 tablespoon coconut oil
- 2 cups onion, chopped
- 2-3 jalapeños or to taste, chopped
- 2 tablespoons garlic, minced
- 2 teaspoons red pepper flakes
- ½ cup fresh cilantro, chopped
- Salt to taste
- Pepper to taste
- 1 cup tomatoes, chopped
- 1 teaspoon ground cumin
- 4 sprigs thyme

Method:

1. Place a skillet over medium heat. Add oil. When the oil is heated, add garlic and sauté until fragrant.

2. Add onions and sauté for a couple of minutes until translucent. Add tomatoes, jalapeño, thyme sprigs and red pepper flakes and sauté for 4-5 minutes.

3. Add turkey and sauté until brown. Break the turkey simultaneously as it cooks.

4. Add salt and pepper and stir.

5. Add cilantro and stir.

6. Serve hot.

Chapter 9: Meal Prep Desserts Recipes

Avocado Chocolate Mousse

Serves: 4

Ingredients:

- 2 large ripe avocado
- 4 tablespoons maple syrup or honey
- 4 tablespoons almond milk
- 8 tablespoons cocoa powder
- 20 drops of liquid stevia or 2 tablespoons of syrup or honey
- Cacao nibs or coconut flakes or strawberries, optional

Methods:

1. Mix all the ingredients in blender until it becomes smooth and creamy.
2. Allow it to freeze before serving.
3. Serve it in a bowl or wine glass, garnished with desired toppings.
4. It can be kept in the refrigerator for 2-3 days.

Chocolate Chia Pudding

Serves: 2

Ingredients:

- 2 Tablespoons chia seeds
- 6 tablespoons milk
- Coconut flakes, cacao nibs or berries, optional
- 2 Tablespoons cocoa powder
- 20 drops of liquid stevia or 2 or more tablespoons of honey

Method:

1. Take a container or a jar and add all the ingredients to it.
2. Now using a fork whisk until the chia seeds get immersed in the liquid properly.
3. Taste to make sure the sweetness of the mixture is to your liking or add more according to your taste buds.
4. Keep it overnight in the fridge or for a minimum of 12 hours for the best results.
5. Serve when required.
6. It can last for 2-3 days in the refrigerator.

Vegan Coconut Oil Chocolates

Yield: 6-8

Ingredients:

- ¼ cup melted coconut oil
- 1 tablespoon mesquite powder
- 1/8 cup toasted almonds
- 1/8 cup raw cacao powder
- 1 tablespoon maple syrup
- 1/8 cup shredded or flaked coconut

Method:

1. Add coconut oil, cacao powder, mesquite powder and maple syrup in a bowl and incorporate well until combined. Take half of the quantity of almonds and coconut and add to this mixture and fold. Rest of the almonds and coconut can be used for garnishing.

2. Take 6-8 small cupcake liners and place in a baking pan. Add mixture to these cupcake liners and garnish with rest of the almonds and coconuts.

3. Cool it in a refrigerator for around 2 hours before serving.

4. Can be stored in the refrigerator for up to a week and served as and when required.

Fresh Berries with Yogurt and Chocolate

Serves: 4

Ingredients:

- 1 basket fresh strawberries
- 1 basket fresh raspberries
- 4 ounce dark chocolate, melted in a double boiler
- 16 ounce low fat vanilla yogurt

Method:

1. Mix berries in a large bowl. Add yogurt and fold gently.
2. Serve berries along with yogurt in individual bowls. Drizzle melted chocolate over it and serve.

Vegan Chocolate Peanut Butter Ice Cream

Serves: 8

Ingredients:

- 4 big bananas, frozen and sliced
- 4 tablespoons creamy natural peanut butter
- ½ teaspoon cinnamon
- 4 tablespoons cocoa powder
- 1 teaspoon vanilla
- 1-2 pinches of salt

Method:

1. Add all the ingredients in a food processor and pulse slowly around 15 seconds at a time until smooth and creamy.

2. It can be frozen in an airtight container for up to 5 days or served immediately.

Triple Coconut Cream Pie

Serves: 8

Ingredients:

For The Custard:

- 4 eggs
- 1 cup sugar
- 1 cup skim milk
- ½ teaspoon vanilla extract
- ½ cup flour
- 1-2 pinches of salt
- 2-13.5 ounce can of light coconut milk

For The Coconut Whipped Cream:

- 2-13.5 ounce can of coconut milk, refrigerated
- 4tablespoons confectioner's sugar
- 1 teaspoon vanilla extract

For the Pie:

- 2 prebaked pie crust
- 6 tablespoons toasted coconut

Method:

To Prepare Custard:

1. Add eggs, flour, sugar and salt in a big bowl. Wisk together and set aside.

2. Take a big saucepan add skim milk and coconut milk. Cook over low heat until it starts to bubble along side of pan. Remove from heat. Pour milk in to the mixture whisking quickly all the while. Now pour this mixture back into the saucepan and place it over a low heat. Let it simmer for about 10-12 minutes until thick and bubbly.

3. Once the mixture thickens take it off from the heat and transfer to a heatproof bowl. Freeze it until the custard is room temperature. Add vanilla extract.

To Prepare the Coconut Whipped Cream:

1. Spoon out the top cream portion of the refrigerated coconut cream into a mixer. Wisk on high for around 3-4 minutes until stiff peaks are formed. Add vanilla and confectioner's sugar.

To assemble the Pie:

1. Now pour the cooled custard into crust. Garnish with whipped cream and toasted coconut. Cover with cling film and freeze for around 6 hours until the custard is chilled.

Carrot Cake Energy Bites

Serves: 20

Ingredients:

- ½ cup walnuts
- 12 medjool dates, pitted
- ½ cup finely shredded coconut + extra to top
- 1 cup carrots, finely grated + extra to top
- ¼ teaspoon sea salt
- 1 teaspoon ground nutmeg

Method:

1. Add dates, ½ cup carrots, coconut, salt and nutmeg into a food processor and pulse until smooth.

2. Add remaining carrots and walnuts and pulse until you get a coarse texture with the nuts visible.

3. Transfer into a bowl. Divide and shape into 20 balls. Roll each in extra shredded coconut and place on a lined baking sheet. Garnish with carrots and serve.

4. Refrigerate the balls until ready to serve.

5. Keep the unused ones refrigerated. It can last for 4-5 days when refrigerated.

Fudgy Skillet Brownie

Serves: 8-10

Ingredients:

- 8 tablespoons coconut oil
- 4 tablespoons mashed ripe banana
- 2 teaspoon vanilla extract
- 2/3 tapioca flour
- 2 cups dark chocolate chips
- Chocolate chips for topping, optional
- ½ teaspoon salt
- 4 eggs
- 3 teaspoon coconut flour

Method:

1. Take a bowl and add coconut oil and chocolate chips to it. Melt and stir until well mixed.
2. Add mashed banana, salt and vanilla and stir.
3. Wisk in the eggs one by one.
4. Mix the flours in this mixture until it just combines.
5. Transfer this mixture in a greased cast iron skillet. Garnish with chocolate chips. Bake for around 22-24 minutes in oven preheated to 350 degrees until it starts to leave the sides and the middle is slightly soft.

Conclusion

I thank you once again for choosing this book and hope you had a good time reading it.

We have done our bit by educating you on the meaning, importance and method of prepping for meals. It is now entirely up to you to prep meals in advance and make it easier for yourself. I hope you put the advice to good use and prepare healthy meals for you and your family.

You need not stick to the recipes mentioned in this book and can come up with some of your own.

Bon Appetit!

THANK YOU! ☺

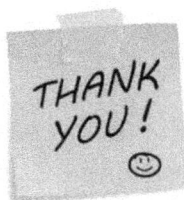

Finally, if you enjoyed this book, then I'd like to ask you for a favor, would you be kind enough to leave a review for this book on Amazon? It'd be greatly appreciated!

Click here to leave a review for this book on Amazon!

Thank you and good luck!

Check Out My Other Books

Below you'll find some of my other popular books that are popular on Amazon and Kindle as well. Simply click on the links below to check them out. Alternatively, you can visit my author page on Amazon to see other work done by me.

CrossFit: Barbell and Dumbbell Exercises for Body Strength

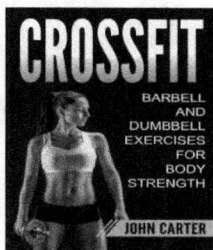

Mediterranean Diet: Step By Step Guide And Proven Recipes For Smart Eating And Weight Loss

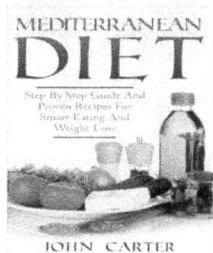

Weight Watchers: Smart Points Cookbook - Step By Step Guide And Proven Recipes For Effective Weight Loss

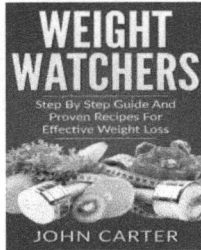

Bodybuilding: Beginners Handbook - Proven Step By Step Guide To Get The Body You Always Dreamed About

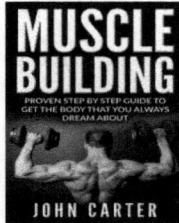

South Beach Diet: Lose Weight and Get Healthy the South Beach Way

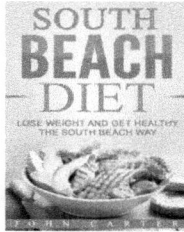

Blood Pressure: Step By Step Guide And Proven Recipes To Lower Your Blood Pressure Without Any Medication

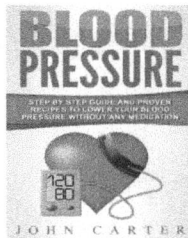

If the links do not work, for whatever reason, you can simply search for these titles on the Amazon website to find them.

www.ingramcontent.com/pod-product-compliance
Lightning Source LLC
Chambersburg PA
CBHW071234020426
42333CB00015B/1466